What in the Perimenopause is this!

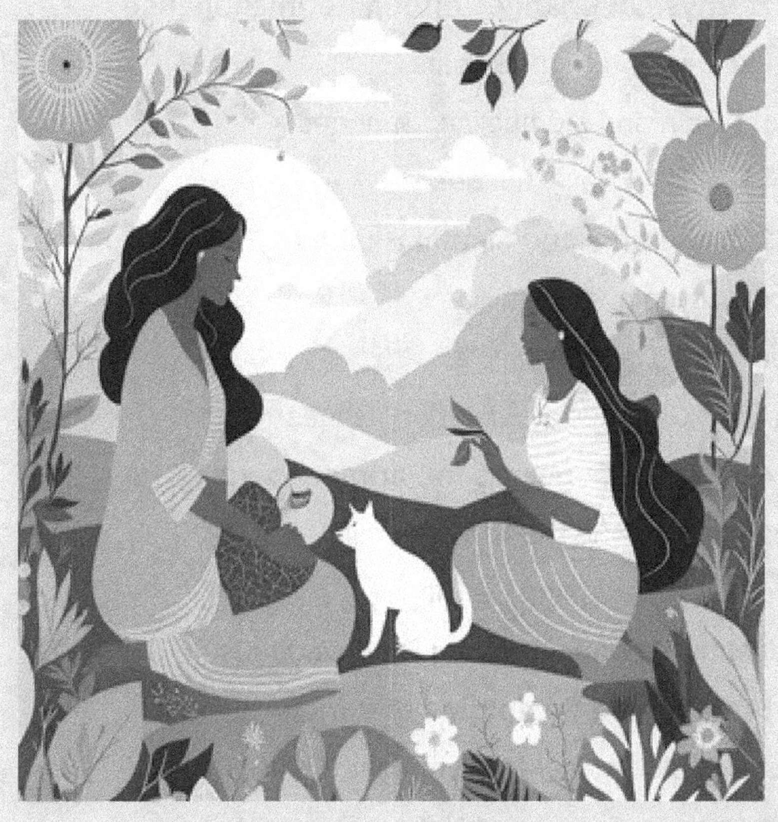

Summary

Chapter 1: Understanding Perimenopause

Chapter 2: Physical Changes during Perimenopause

Chapter 3: Emotional and Mental Health in Perimenopause

Chapter 4: Fertility Concerns in Perimenopause

Chapter 5: Managing Symptoms of Perimenopause

Chapter 6: Navigating Relationships and Communication in Perimenopause

Chapter 1: Understanding Perimenopause

1.1 The Definition and Duration of Perimenopause

Perimenopause, often referred to as the menopausal transition, is a natural phase in a woman's life that typically begins in her 40s but can start earlier for some women. It is characterized by hormonal fluctuations and changes that signal the approach of menopause, which marks the end of a woman's reproductive years. Unlike menopause, which is defined as the cessation of menstruation for 12 consecutive months, perimenopause involves irregular menstrual cycles and various symptoms that can last for several years before menopause officially occurs.

During perimenopause, the ovaries gradually produce less estrogen and progesterone, leading to hormonal imbalances that can impact a woman's physical and emotional well-being. These hormonal shifts can result in a range of symptoms such as hot flashes, night sweats, mood swings, fatigue, insomnia, vaginal dryness, and changes in libido. While each woman's experience with perimenopause is unique, these common symptoms are often disruptive and challenging to manage without proper support and understanding.

The duration of perimenopause varies for each individual but typically lasts around four to eight years before menopause is reached. However, some women may experience a shorter or longer transition period depending on factors such as genetics, lifestyle choices, overall health status, and medical history. It is essential for women to recognize the signs of perimenopause early on so they can proactively address any concerns or seek appropriate medical guidance to navigate this transformative phase with greater ease.

Understanding the definition and duration of perimenopause is crucial for women approaching this life stage as it prepares them for the changes ahead and empowers them to take control of their health and well-being during this transitional period.

1.2 Hormonal Changes and Fluctuations

Hormonal changes play a significant role in driving the symptoms experienced during perimenopause. As women age, their ovaries produce less estrogen and progesterone, leading to imbalances that can trigger a cascade of physical and emotional effects. Estrogen levels fluctuate unpredictably during perimenopause, causing irregular menstrual cycles, hot flashes, night sweats, mood swings, and other symptoms that vary in intensity from woman to woman.

Progesterone levels also decline during perimenopause, affecting the regulation of the menstrual cycle and contributing to symptoms like insomnia, anxiety, irritability, and breast tenderness. These hormonal fluctuations can disrupt the body's internal balance and impact various systems such as metabolism, bone density maintenance...

Moreover...

For further reading on perimenopause and hormonal changes, consider exploring resources such as "The Wisdom of Menopause" by Dr. Christiane Northrup, "The Hormone Cure" by Dr. Sara Gottfried, or articles from reputable sources like the Mayo Clinic or Harvard Health Publishing. These sources provide valuable insights into understanding the hormonal shifts that occur during perimenopause and offer practical tips for managing symptoms and optimizing health during this transitional phase.

Chapter 2: Physical Changes during Perimenopause

2.1 Hot Flashes and Night Sweats

Hot flashes and night sweats are common symptoms experienced by women during perimenopause. These sudden feelings of intense heat, often accompanied by sweating, can be disruptive and uncomfortable. While the exact cause of hot flashes is not fully understood, hormonal fluctuations, particularly a decrease in estrogen levels, are believed to play a significant role.

For many women, hot flashes can occur multiple times throughout the day and night, leading to sleep disturbances and overall decreased quality of life. The unpredictability of these episodes can also impact social interactions and daily activities. Managing hot flashes may involve lifestyle changes such as wearing breathable clothing, maintaining a cool environment, practicing relaxation techniques like deep breathing or meditation, and avoiding triggers like spicy foods or caffeine.

It is essential for women experiencing hot flashes to communicate openly with their healthcare provider to explore treatment options that may include hormone therapy or other medications. Additionally, engaging in regular exercise, maintaining a healthy weight, and prioritizing self-care practices can help alleviate the frequency and intensity of hot flashes.

Real-life experiences shared by women going through perimenopause can shed light on the diverse ways in which individuals cope with hot flashes. Some may find relief through alternative therapies like acupuncture or herbal supplements, while others may rely on prescription medications for symptom management. Understanding that each woman's journey through perimenopause is unique can foster empathy and support within communities facing similar challenges.

2.2 Weight Gain and Metabolism Changes

Weight gain and metabolism changes are common concerns for women entering perimenopause. Fluctuations in hormone levels can impact how the body stores fat and processes energy, leading to an increase in abdominal fat deposition and a decrease in muscle mass. These changes can contribute to weight gain, especially around the midsection.

Metabolism naturally slows down with age, but hormonal shifts during perimenopause can further exacerbate this process. Women may notice that they have to work harder to maintain their weight or that weight loss becomes more challenging than before. Adopting a balanced diet rich in fruits, vegetables, lean proteins, and whole grains while limiting processed foods and sugary beverages can support metabolic health during this transitional phase.

Regular physical activity is crucial for managing weight gain and supporting overall well-being during perimenopause. Incorporating strength training exercises to preserve muscle mass, along with cardiovascular activities like walking or swimming to boost metabolism, can help offset the effects of hormonal changes on body composition.

Women navigating weight gain during perimenopause may benefit from seeking guidance from healthcare professionals such as nutritionists or personal trainers who specialize in menopausal health. By developing personalized strategies tailored to individual needs and goals, women can proactively address weight management challenges while promoting long-term health outcomes.

Sharing success stories of women who have embraced lifestyle modifications to combat weight gain during perimenopause can inspire others facing similar struggles. From adopting mindful eating habits to finding joy in physical movement routines, these narratives highlight the resilience and determination exhibited by individuals taking charge of their health amidst hormonal transitions. 2.3 Skin, Hair, and Nail Changes Perimenopause can bring about various changes in skin elasticity, hair texture, and nail strength that may come as a surprise to some women.

The decline in estrogen levels can lead to reduced collagen production, resulting in thinner skin and increased dryness. These changes may manifest as fine lines, wrinkles, and sagging skin. Therefore, women may need to reevaluate their skincare routines and seek products that promote hydration and rejuvenation. Hair thinning or loss is another common concern during perimenopause, as hormonal imbalances can affect hair growth cycles. Women may notice increased shedding, changes in hair texture, or even bald patches, which can impact self-esteem and confidence. To mitigate these effects and promote regrowth, women can explore hair care options such as gentle shampoos, scalp treatments, or dietary supplements rich in vitamins and minerals essential for hair health. Nail changes, such as brittleness, ridges, or slow growth rates, are also prevalent among women experiencing perimenopause. Hormonal fluctuations can weaken nails, but proper nail care practices can help improve their health. These practices include moisturizing cuticles, using strengthening treatments, and avoiding harsh chemicals found in some nail products. Women can also incorporate biotin-rich foods into their diets or consider oral supplements recommended by healthcare providers to further support nail health.

  that may catch some women off guard. The decline in estrogen levels can lead to reduced collagen production, resulting in thinner skin and increased dryness. These shifts may manifest as fine lines, wrinkles, and sagging skin, prompting individuals to reassess their skincare routines and seek products that promote hydration and rejuvenation.

  Hair thinning or loss is another common concern during perimenopause, as hormonal imbalances can affect hair growth cycles. Women may notice increased shedding, changes in hair texture, or even bald patches, which can impact self-esteem and confidence. Exploring hair care options such as gentle shampoos, scalp treatments, or dietary supplements rich in vitamins and minerals essential for hair health may help mitigate these effects and promote regrowth.

Nail changes, such as brittleness, ridges, or slow growth rates, are also prevalent among women experiencing perimenopause. The weakening of nails due to hormonal fluctuations can be addressed through proper nail care practices like moisturizing cuticles, using strengthening treatments, and avoiding harsh chemicals found in some nail products. Incorporating biotin-rich foods into one's diet or considering oral supplements recommended by healthcare providers

By sharing personal anecdotes about navigating skin concerns during perimenopause—whether it's discovering new skincare routines that enhance radiance or seeking professional advice for specific dermatological issues—women can empower each other with knowledge and encouragement to embrace their changing bodies with confidence and grace. Through open conversations about skin care challenges during this transitional phase of life women can build supportive networks that prioritize self-care and well-being amidst physical transformations

For further reading on managing symptoms of perimenopause, including hot flashes, weight gain, and skin changes, consider exploring reputable sources such as the North American Menopause Society (NAMS) website (www.menopause.org) or the Mayo Clinic's resources on menopause (www.mayoclinic.org). Additionally, books like "The Menopause Solution" by Dr. Stephanie Faubion or "Menopause Confidential" by Dr. Tara Allmen offer valuable insights and practical advice for navigating this life stage with confidence and empowerment.

Chapter 3: Emotional and Mental Health in Perimenopause

Perimenopause is a phase of significant hormonal changes, especially a decrease in estrogen levels, which can impact a woman's emotional well-being. Mood swings and irritability are common symptoms experienced during this time, often leaving women feeling overwhelmed and emotionally unstable. Although the exact mechanisms behind mood swings and irritability in perimenopause are not fully understood, it is believed that hormonal imbalances play a crucial role in disrupting neurotransmitter activity in the brain. This disruption can lead to sudden shifts in mood, ranging from feelings of sadness and anxiety to anger and frustration. The unpredictability of these emotional changes can be challenging to navigate, both for the individual experiencing them and those around them. Real-life experiences shared by women going through perimenopause highlight the various ways individuals cope with mood swings and irritability. Some find comfort in mindfulness practices such as meditation or yoga, while others may seek therapy or support groups to process their emotions effectively. Understanding that these emotional changes are a natural part of the menopausal transition can help women feel less alone in their struggles.

It is essential for women experiencing severe mood swings or irritability to communicate openly with their healthcare provider to explore treatment options that may include therapy, medication, or hormone replacement therapy. Additionally, adopting self-care practices such as regular exercise, adequate sleep, healthy eating habits, and stress management techniques can help regulate emotions and improve overall mental well-being during perimenopause.

By sharing personal anecdotes about navigating mood swings and irritability during perimenopause—whether it's finding comfort in creative outlets like art or music therapy or practicing relaxation techniques like deep breathing exercises—women can empower each other with strategies for managing their emotional health effectively. Building a supportive network of friends, family members, or healthcare professionals who understand and validate these experiences can make a significant difference in how women navigate this challenging phase of life.

3.2 Anxiety and Depression

Anxiety and depression are prevalent mental health concerns that can arise during perimenopause due to hormonal fluctuations and other factors associated with this stage of life. Women may experience heightened feelings of worry, fear, restlessness, or sadness that interfere with daily functioning and overall quality of life.

It is essential for women experiencing severe mood swings or irritability to communicate openly with their healthcare provider to explore treatment options that may include therapy, medication, or hormone replacement therapy. Additionally, adopting self-care practices such as regular exercise, adequate sleep, healthy eating habits, and stress management techniques can help regulate emotions and improve overall mental well-being during perimenopause.

By sharing personal anecdotes about navigating mood swings and irritability during perimenopause—whether it's finding comfort in creative outlets like art or music therapy or practicing relaxation techniques like deep breathing exercises—women can empower each other with strategies for managing their emotional health effectively. Building a supportive network of friends, family members, or healthcare professionals who understand and validate these experiences can make a significant difference in how women navigate this challenging phase of life.

3.2 Anxiety and Depression

Anxiety and depression are common mental health concerns that can arise during perimenopause due to hormonal fluctuations and other factors associated with this stage of life. Women may experience heightened feelings of worry, fear, restlessness, or sadness that can interfere with daily functioning and overall quality of life. The hormonal changes occurring during perimenopause can impact neurotransmitter activity in the brain, leading to imbalances that contribute to symptoms of anxiety and depression. Additionally, factors such as stress, lifestyle changes, sleep disturbances, and underlying psychological issues can worsen these mental health conditions during this transitional phase.

It is essential for women experiencing severe anxiety or depression symptoms during perimenopause to seek professional help from therapists, counselors, or psychiatrists. Cognitive-behavioral therapy (CBT) or medication prescribed by healthcare providers can provide effective tools for managing these mental health challenges. To support their mental well-being during this period of change, women should prioritize self-care practices like regular exercise, adequate sleep, healthy eating, and stress management techniques.

Real-life stories shared by women navigating anxiety and depression during perimenopause can shed light on the resilience and strength exhibited by individuals facing mental health struggles. Some may find relief through holistic approaches like acupuncture, meditation, or herbal supplements,

while others may benefit from traditional therapies such as antidepressants or anti-anxiety medications. Understanding that seeking help is a sign of strength and courage can empower women to take control of their mental health and seek support when needed.

By fostering open conversations about anxiety and depression during perimenopause—whether it's discussing coping strategies with loved ones or sharing resources for mental health support—women can create a safe space for addressing these sensitive topics. Building a community that prioritizes mental well-being and destigmatizes discussions around anxiety and depression can promote healing and resilience among individuals navigating this challenging phase of life.

3.3 Cognitive Changes and Memory Issues

Cognitive changes and memory issues are common concerns faced by women entering perimenopause, as hormonal fluctuations can impact brain function and cognitive abilities. Women may notice difficulties with concentration, memory recall, or multitasking tasks they once found effortless, leading to feelings of frustration and cognitive decline.

Research indicates that estrogen hormone is crucial for supporting neuronal function and synaptic plasticity within the brain. However, during the ageing process, estrogen levels decline, which may lead to disruptions in neurotransmitter activity. This disruption can have an impact on cognitive processes such as attention, memory encoding, and executive function in women.

Real-life experiences shared by women going through perimenopause highlight the diverse ways individuals cope with cognitive changes and memory issues. Some may implement memory-enhancing strategies like mnemonic devices or daily routines to support cognitive function, while others may seek professional guidance from neuropsychologists or cognitive therapists for tailored interventions. Understanding that cognitive changes are a normal part of aging but also influenced by hormonal shifts during menopause can help women approach these challenges with compassion towards themselves.

Engaging in activities that stimulate brain health such as puzzles, reading, learning new skills, or socializing with others can promote cognitive resilience during perimenopause.

Additionally, adopting lifestyle habits known to support brain function such as regular physical exercise,

By fostering open conversations about anxiety and depression during perimenopause—whether it's discussing coping strategies with loved ones or sharing resources for mental health support—women can create a safe space for addressing these sensitive topics. Building a community that prioritizes mental well-being and destigmatizes discussions around anxiety and depression can promote healing and resilience among individuals navigating this challenging phase of life.

3.3 Cognitive Changes and Memory Issues

Cognitive changes and memory issues are common concerns faced by women entering perimenopause, as hormonal fluctuations can impact brain function and cognitive abilities. Women may notice difficulties with concentration, memory recall, or multitasking tasks they once found effortless, leading to feelings of frustration and cognitive decline.

Research indicates that estrogen hormone is crucial for supporting neuronal function and synaptic plasticity within the brain. However, during the ageing process, estrogen levels decline, which may lead to disruptions in neurotransmitter activity. This disruption can have an impact on cognitive processes such as attention, memory encoding, and executive function in women.

Real-life experiences shared by women going through perimenopause highlight the diverse ways individuals cope with cognitive changes and memory issues. Some may implement memory-enhancing strategies like mnemonic devices or daily routines to support cognitive function, while others may seek professional guidance from neuropsychologists or cognitive therapists for tailored interventions. Understanding that cognitive changes are a normal part of aging but also influenced by hormonal shifts during menopause can help women approach these challenges with compassion towards themselves.

Engaging in activities that stimulate brain health such as puzzles, reading, learning new skills, or socializing with others can promote cognitive resilience during perimenopause.

It's important to adopt lifestyle habits that support brain function, especially during the transitional phase of perimenopause. This includes regular physical exercise, a balanced diet rich in antioxidants, omega-3 fatty acids, vitamins and minerals, adequate sleep, and stress management techniques. These practices can enhance overall cognitive well-being and help manage memory issues. Women who experience significant cognitive changes during this phase should communicate openly with healthcare providers to explore potential treatment options such as hormone therapy, cognitive training programs, or medications that target specific cognitive deficits. Sharing personal anecdotes about navigating cognitive changes can help empower other women with practical tips for maintaining cognitive vitality amidst hormonal transitions. Building a supportive network of peers, family members, or healthcare professionals who understand the challenges associated with cognitive changes can provide valuable encouragement and validation for individuals navigating this aspect of menopausal transition.

but research suggests that estrogen plays a crucial role in supporting neuronal function and synaptic plasticity within the brain. As estrogen levels decline during this stage of life, women may experience disruptions in neurotransmitter activity, which can affect cognitive processes such as attention, memory encoding, and executive function.

Real-life experiences shared by women going through perimenopause highlight the diverse ways individuals cope with cognitive changes and memory issues. Some may implement memory-enhancing strategies like mnemonic devices or daily routines to support cognitive function, while others may seek professional guidance from neuropsychologists or cognitive therapists for tailored interventions. Understanding that cognitive changes are a normal part of aging but also influenced by hormonal shifts during menopause can help women approach these challenges with compassion towards themselves.

Engaging in activities that stimulate brain health, such as solving puzzles, diving into a good book, learning new skills, or connecting with others socially, can play a significant role in boosting cognitive resilience during perimenopause. Alongside these activities, incorporating lifestyle habits that are known to support brain function, like engaging in regular physical exercise,

It is crucial for women facing intense mood swings or irritability to have open conversations with their healthcare provider to explore various treatment options. These options may include therapy, medication, or hormone replacement therapy. Furthermore, embracing self-care practices such as maintaining a consistent exercise routine, getting enough restful sleep, following a nutritious diet, and utilizing stress management techniques can effectively help in regulating emotions and enhancing overall mental well-being throughout perimenopause.

Have you ever tried challenging your brain with puzzles or new skills during perimenopause? How did it make you feel? Share your experience!

It is essential for women experiencing severe mood swings or irritability to communicate openly with their healthcare provider to explore treatment options that may include therapy, medication, or hormone replacement therapy. Additionally, adopting self-care practices such as regular exercise, adequate sleep, healthy eating habits, and stress management techniques can help regulate emotions and improve overall mental well-being during perimenopause.

By sharing personal anecdotes about navigating mood swings and irritability during perimenopause—whether it's finding comfort in creative outlets like art or music therapy or practicing relaxation techniques like deep breathing exercises—women can empower each other with strategies for managing their emotional health effectively. Building a supportive network of friends, family members, or healthcare professionals who understand and validate these experiences can make a significant difference in how women navigate this challenging phase of life.

3.2 Anxiety and Depression

Anxiety and depression are common mental health concerns that can arise during perimenopause due to hormonal fluctuations and other factors associated with this stage of life. Women may experience heightened feelings of worry, fear, restlessness, or sadness that can interfere with daily functioning and overall quality of life. The hormonal changes occurring during perimenopause can impact neurotransmitter activity in the brain, leading to imbalances that contribute to symptoms of anxiety and depression. Additionally, factors such as stress, lifestyle changes, sleep disturbances, and underlying psychological issues can worsen these mental health conditions during this transitional phase.

It is essential for women experiencing severe anxiety or depression symptoms during perimenopause to seek professional help from therapists, counselors, or psychiatrists. Cognitive-behavioral therapy (CBT) or medication prescribed by healthcare providers can provide effective tools for managing these mental health challenges. To support their mental well-being during this period of change, women should prioritize self-care practices like regular exercise, adequate sleep, healthy eating, and stress management techniques.

Real-life stories shared by women navigating anxiety and depression during perimenopause can shed light on the resilience and strength exhibited by individuals facing mental health struggles. Some may find relief through holistic approaches like acupuncture, meditation, or herbal supplements,

while others may benefit from traditional therapies such as antidepressants or anti-anxiety medications. Understanding that seeking help is a sign of strength and courage can empower women to take control of their mental health and seek support when needed.

By fostering open conversations about anxiety and depression during perimenopause—whether it's discussing coping strategies with loved ones or sharing resources for mental health support—women can create a safe space for addressing these sensitive topics. Building a community that prioritizes mental well-being and destigmatizes discussions around anxiety and depression can promote healing and resilience among individuals navigating this challenging phase of life.

3.3 Cognitive Changes and Memory Issues

Cognitive changes and memory issues are common concerns faced by women entering perimenopause, as hormonal fluctuations can impact brain function and cognitive abilities. Women may notice difficulties with concentration, memory recall, or multitasking tasks they once found effortless, leading to feelings of frustration and cognitive decline.

Research indicates that estrogen hormone is crucial for supporting neuronal function and synaptic plasticity within the brain. However, during the ageing process, estrogen levels decline, which may lead to disruptions in neurotransmitter activity. This disruption can have an impact on cognitive processes such as attention, memory encoding, and executive function in women.

Real-life experiences shared by women going through perimenopause highlight the diverse ways individuals cope with cognitive changes and memory issues. Some may implement memory-enhancing strategies like mnemonic devices or daily routines to support cognitive function, while others may seek professional guidance from neuropsychologists or cognitive therapists for tailored interventions. Understanding that cognitive changes are a normal part of aging but also influenced by hormonal shifts during menopause can help women approach these challenges with compassion towards themselves.

Engaging in activities that stimulate brain health such as puzzles, reading, learning new skills, or socializing with others can promote cognitive resilience during perimenopause.

It's important to adopt lifestyle habits that support brain function, especially during the transitional phase of perimenopause. This includes regular physical exercise, a balanced diet rich in antioxidants, omega-3 fatty acids, vitamins and minerals, adequate sleep, and stress management techniques. These practices can enhance overall cognitive well-being and help manage memory issues. Women who experience significant cognitive changes during this phase should communicate openly with healthcare providers to explore potential treatment options such as hormone therapy, cognitive training programs, or medications that target specific cognitive deficits. Sharing personal anecdotes about navigating cognitive changes can help empower other women with practical tips for maintaining cognitive vitality amidst hormonal transitions. Building a supportive network of peers, family members, or healthcare professionals who understand the challenges associated with cognitive changes can provide valuable encouragement and validation for individuals navigating this aspect of menopausal transition.

For further reading on managing mood swings, anxiety, depression, cognitive changes, and memory issues during perimenopause, consider exploring the following resources:

1."The Wisdom of Menopause: Creating Physical and Emotional Health During the Change" by Christiane Northrup, M.D.

2."Menopause Confidential: A Doctor Reveals the Secrets to Thriving Through Midlife" by Tara Allmen, MD

3."The Hormone Cure: Reclaim Balance, Sleep and Sex Drive; Lose Weight; Feel Focused, Vital, and Energized Naturally with the Gottfried Protocol" by Sara Gottfried, MD

These books offer valuable insights and practical strategies for navigating the challenges of perimenopause with a focus on emotional well-being and cognitive health.

Chapter 4: Fertility Concerns in Perimenopause

4.1 Understanding the Decline in Fertility

As women approach perimenopause, their fertility tends to decline due to biological factors. Knowing about these factors can help them make informed decisions about family planning and explore alternative options if they wish to preserve their fertility. Therefore, it is crucial for women at this stage of life to consult with their healthcare providers or fertility specialists to evaluate their reproductive health and discuss potential strategies for conceiving if they desire.

While women are born with a finite number of eggs that steadily decrease over time, the quality of these eggs also diminishes as they age. This decline in egg quality can impact fertilization rates, embryo development, and overall pregnancy success. Additionally, hormonal changes during perimenopause can disrupt the regular ovulation cycle, making it more challenging to conceive naturally.

Understanding the causes of declining fertility during perimenopause can help women make informed decisions about family planning and explore alternative options if they wish to preserve their fertility. It is essential for women approaching this stage of life to consult with healthcare providers or fertility specialists to assess their reproductive health and discuss potential strategies for conceiving if desired.

For further reading on fertility preservation options, pregnancy during perimenopause, and navigating reproductive health challenges, consider exploring resources such as "The Fertility Handbook: A Guide to Getting Pregnant" by Dr. Mark Trolice, "Expecting Better: Why the Conventional Pregnancy Wisdom Is Wrong--and What You Really Need to Know" by Emily Oster, and "Taking Charge of Your Fertility" by Toni Weschler. Additionally, consulting reputable medical websites like the American

Society for Reproductive Medicine (ASRM) or the Mayo Clinic can provide valuable information on reproductive health topics.

For further reading on fertility preservation options, pregnancy during perimenopause, and navigating reproductive health challenges, consider exploring resources such as "The Fertility Handbook: A Guide to Getting Pregnant" by Dr. Mark Trolice, "Expecting Better: Why the Conventional Pregnancy Wisdom Is Wrong--and What You Really Need to Know" by Emily Oster, and "Taking Charge of Your Fertility" by Toni Weschler. Additionally, consulting reputable medical websites like the American Society for Reproductive Medicine (ASRM) or the Mayo Clinic can provide valuable information on reproductive health topics.

One common approach to preserving fertility during perimenopause is through egg freezing, a process that involves retrieving mature eggs from the ovaries, freezing them for future use, and later thawing them when ready to conceive. Egg freezing allows women to safeguard their reproductive capacity by storing healthy eggs at a younger age when they are most viable for fertilization.

Another option for preserving fertility is embryo cryopreservation, where eggs are fertilized with sperm from a partner or donor before being frozen as embryos. This method offers an additional layer of security by ensuring that embryos are already formed and ready for implantation when desired pregnancy occurs.

For women who may not have viable eggs due to age-related factors or medical conditions affecting ovarian function, using donor eggs or embryos presents an alternative solution for achieving pregnancy. Donor-assisted reproduction provides individuals with the opportunity to experience pregnancy and childbirth while overcoming infertility challenges related to advanced maternal age.

Exploring these various options for preserving fertility empowers women with choices regarding their reproductive futures during perimenopause. By consulting with fertility specialists or reproductive endocrinologists, individuals can gain insights into personalized treatment plans tailored to their unique needs and preferences. Open discussions about ethical considerations,

financial implications, and emotional readiness for pursuing assisted reproduction can help individuals make well-informed decisions about which path aligns best with their values and goals.

Real-life stories shared by women who have undergone fertility preservation treatments offer insights into the emotional journey of navigating these complex decisions. Some may find solace in connecting with others who have faced similar challenges, while others may seek guidance from mental health professionals to process feelings of uncertainty or grief surrounding infertility. By fostering open conversations about fertility preservation options, women can create a supportive community that normalizes discussions around reproductive health and empowers individuals to take control of their family-building aspirations.

4.3 Navigating Pregnancy during Perimenopause

Pregnancy during perimenopause presents a myriad of unique considerations and challenges due to age-related factors that significantly impact maternal health, foetal development, and overall pregnancy outcomes. While the possibility of conception still exists during this transitional phase, it is crucial for women to be cognizant of the potential risks associated with advanced maternal age and actively engage in discussions with healthcare providers to ensure they receive optimal prenatal care.

Navigating pregnancy amidst perimenopause demands a heightened awareness of the intricate interplay between aging processes and reproductive health. Women embarking on this journey must grapple with a complex tapestry of physiological changes that can influence the course of their pregnancy. The dynamic nature of perimenopause introduces a layer of complexity that necessitates a tailored approach to prenatal care.

Maternal health considerations take centre stage as women traverse the delicate balance between menopausal symptoms and the demands of pregnancy. The physiological shifts inherent in perimenopause can pose challenges such as hormonal imbalances, which may impact fertility and gestational well-being. It is imperative for women to proactively address these age-related factors through proactive consultations with healthcare professionals.

Foetal development also assumes heightened significance in pregnancies occurring during perimenopause. The aging process can potentially affect the quality of eggs, leading to an increased risk of chromosomal abnormalities and other developmental issues. This underscores the importance of vigilant monitoring and specialized interventions to optimize foetal growth and mitigate potential complications.

Overall pregnancy outcomes are intricately intertwined with age-related considerations that underscore the need for comprehensive care strategies tailored to the unique needs of women navigating pregnancy during perimenopause. By fostering open communication with healthcare providers, women can access a wealth of resources aimed at promoting maternal well-being and ensuring positive pregnancy experiences despite the challenges posed by advanced maternal age.

In essence, embracing the journey of pregnancy during perimenopause entails a nuanced understanding of age-related factors that shape maternal health, foetal development, and overall pregnancy outcomes. Through proactive engagement with healthcare providers and a commitment to personalized care approaches, women can navigate this transformative phase with resilience and empowerment, ultimately paving the way for healthy pregnancies amidst the complexities of perimenopause.

Women experiencing unexpected pregnancies during perimenopause should seek early prenatal care to monitor maternal health and foetal development closely. Healthcare providers may recommend additional screenings or tests to assess any potential risks associated with advanced maternal age such as chromosomal abnormalities or gestational diabetes.

Real-life experiences shared by women navigating pregnancies during perimenopause highlight the resilience and adaptability exhibited throughout this transformative journey. Some may find comfort in connecting with other expectant mothers facing similar circumstances while others may seek guidance from obstetricians or maternal-foetal medicine specialists for specialized care.

By prioritizing self-care practices such as proper nutrition, regular exercise, prenatal vitamins, adequate rest, and stress management techniques, women can support their overall well-being during pregnancy in perimenopause. Building a strong support system of partners, family members, friends, and healthcare providers can provide invaluable encouragement and assistance throughout this unique chapter of motherhood. Navigating pregnancy during perimenopause requires careful consideration.

Have you ever wondered how to balance self-care with the demands of pregnancy during perimenopause? What are some effective stress management techniques that have worked for you during this time? Share your experiences with building a support system that has helped you navigate the challenges of motherhood in perimenopause.

 to ensure optimal prenatal care

Women experiencing unexpected pregnancies during perimenopause should seek early prenatal care to monitor maternal health and fetal development closely. Healthcare providers may recommend additional screenings or tests to assess any potential risks associated with advanced maternal age such as chromosomal abnormalities or gestational diabetes.

Real-life experiences shared by women navigating pregnancies during perimenopause highlight the resilience and adaptability exhibited throughout this transformative journey. Some may find comfort in connecting with other expectant mothers facing similar circumstances while others may seek guidance from obstetricians or maternal-fetal medicine specialists for specialized care.

Prioritizing self-care practices such as proper nutrition, regular exercise, prenatal vitamins, adequate rest, and stress management techniques is crucial for women to support their overall well-being during pregnancy in perimenopause. Building a strong support system of partners, family members, friends, and healthcare providers can provide invaluable encouragement and assistance throughout this unique chapter of motherhood.

Navigating pregnancy during perimenopause requires careful consideration. Have you ever thought about how self-care practices can impact your well-being during this special time? What are some ways you can build a strong support system to help you through the challenges of pregnancy in perimenopause? Share your thoughts and experiences with us!

For further reading on fertility preservation options, pregnancy during perimenopause, and navigating reproductive health challenges, consider exploring resources such as "The Fertility Handbook: A Guide to Getting Pregnant" by Dr. Mark Trolice, "Expecting Better: Why the Conventional Pregnancy Wisdom Is Wrong--and What You Really Need to Know" by Emily Oster, and "Taking Charge of Your Fertility" by Toni Weschler. Additionally, consulting reputable medical websites like the American Society for Reproductive Medicine (ASRM) or the Mayo Clinic can provide valuable information on reproductive health topics.

Chapter 5: Managing Symptoms of Perimenopause

5.1 Lifestyle Adjustments for Symptom Relief

Perimenopause can bring about a variety of symptoms such as hot flashes, mood swings, and sleep disturbances that can significantly impact a woman's quality of life. While these symptoms are a natural part of the transition to menopause, there are several lifestyle adjustments that women can make to help alleviate discomfort and improve overall well-being.

One key lifestyle adjustment is maintaining a healthy diet rich in fruits, vegetables, whole grains, and lean proteins. Eating a balanced diet can help regulate hormone levels, manage weight gain often associated with perimenopause, and reduce the frequency and intensity of hot flashes. Additionally, staying hydrated by drinking plenty of water throughout the day can also help alleviate symptoms like dry skin and vaginal dryness.

Regular exercise is another essential component of managing perimenopausal symptoms. Engaging in physical activity such as walking, yoga, or swimming not only helps maintain a healthy weight but also boosts mood, reduces stress levels, and improves sleep quality. Exercise releases endorphins—feel-good hormones—that can counteract feelings of anxiety or depression commonly experienced during this phase.

Incorporating stress management techniques into daily routines can also be beneficial for symptom relief. Practices like mindfulness meditation, deep breathing exercises, or journaling can help women cope with emotional fluctuations and promote relaxation. Prioritizing self-care activities such as taking time for oneself, getting adequate rest, and engaging in hobbies or interests can further enhance overall well-being during perimenopause.

Seeking support from friends, family members, or support groups can provide emotional validation and encouragement during this transitional phase. Connecting with others who are going through similar experiences can create a sense of camaraderie and solidarity that eases feelings of isolation or uncertainty. Additionally, talking to healthcare providers about symptom management strategies or exploring complementary therapies like acupuncture or herbal supplements may offer additional relief for perimenopausal symptoms.

By making intentional lifestyle adjustments tailored to individual needs and preferences, women navigating perimenopause can effectively manage symptoms and enhance their overall quality of life during this transformative stage.

5.2 Alternative Therapies and Natural Remedies

In addition to lifestyle adjustments, alternative therapies and natural remedies can offer additional support for managing perimenopausal symptoms. While hormone replacement therapy (HRT) is a common treatment option, some women may prefer alternative approaches that focus on holistic healing and natural interventions.

One popular alternative therapy for perimenopausal symptom relief is acupuncture, a traditional Chinese medicine practice that involves inserting thin needles into specific points on the body. Acupuncture has been shown to help regulate hormone levels, reduce hot flashes, improve sleep quality, and alleviate mood swings associated with perimenopause.

Herbal supplements such as black cohosh, dong quai, or evening primrose oil are also commonly used to address menopausal symptoms. These botanical remedies contain phytoestrogens—plant-based compounds that mimic estrogen in the body— which may help balance hormone levels and alleviate hot flashes or night sweats.

Mind-body practices like yoga, meditation, or tai chi can promote relaxation, reduce stress levels, and improve overall well-being during perimenopause. These practices focus on connecting the mind, body, and spirit to foster inner peace

Incorporating stress management techniques into daily routines can also be beneficial for symptom relief. Practices like mindfulness meditation, deep breathing exercises, or journaling can help women cope with emotional fluctuations and promote relaxation. Prioritizing self-care activities such as taking time for oneself, getting adequate rest, and engaging in hobbies or interests can further enhance overall well-being during perimenopause.

Seeking support from friends, family members, or support groups can provide emotional validation and encouragement during this transitional phase. Connecting with others who are going through similar experiences can create a sense of camaraderie and solidarity that eases feelings of isolation or uncertainty. Additionally, talking to healthcare providers about symptom management strategies or exploring complementary therapies like acupuncture or herbal supplements may offer additional relief for perimenopausal symptoms.

By making intentional lifestyle adjustments tailored to individual needs and preferences, women navigating perimenopause can effectively manage symptoms and enhance their overall quality of life during this transformative stage.

5.2 Alternative Therapies and Natural Remedies

In addition to lifestyle adjustments, alternative therapies and natural remedies can offer additional support for managing perimenopausal symptoms. While hormone replacement therapy (HRT) is a common treatment option, some women may prefer alternative approaches that focus on holistic healing and natural interventions.

One popular alternative therapy for perimenopausal symptom relief is acupuncture, a traditional Chinese medicine practice that involves inserting thin needles into specific points on the body. Acupuncture has been shown to help regulate hormone levels, reduce hot flashes, improve sleep quality, and alleviate mood swings associated with perimenopause.

Herbal supplements such as black cohosh, dong quai, or evening primrose oil are also commonly used to address menopausal symptoms. These botanical remedies contain phytoestrogens—plant-based compounds that mimic estrogen in the body— which may help balance hormone levels and alleviate hot flashes or night sweats.

Mind-body practices like yoga, meditation, or tai chi can promote relaxation, reduce stress levels, and improve overall well-being during perimenopause. These practices focus on connecting the mind, body, and spirit to foster inner peace

In addition to lifestyle adjustments, alternative therapies and natural remedies can offer additional support for managing perimenopausal symptoms. While hormone replacement therapy (HRT) is a common treatment option, some women may prefer alternative approaches that focus on holistic healing and natural interventions.

One popular alternative therapy for perimenopausal symptom relief is acupuncture, a traditional Chinese medicine practice that involves inserting thin needles into specific points on the body. Acupuncture has been shown to help regulate hormone levels, reduce hot flashes, improve sleep quality, and alleviate mood swings associated with perimenopause.

Herbal supplements such as black cohosh, dong quai, or evening primrose oil are also commonly used to address menopausal symptoms. These botanical remedies contain phytoestrogens—plant-based compounds that mimic estrogen in the body— which may help balance hormone levels and alleviate hot flashes or night sweats.

Mind-body practices like yoga, meditation, or tai chi can promote relaxation, reduce stress levels, and improve overall well-being during perimenopause. These practices focus on connecting the mind, body, and spirit to foster inner peace
and emotional resilience in the face of hormonal changes.

It is suggested that incorporating dietary supplements like vitamin D3, calcium or magnesium in the routine can be beneficial for supporting bone health and reducing the risk of osteoporosis associated with declining estrogen levels during perimenopause. However, before including any alternative therapies or natural remedies in the routine, women should consult with healthcare providers to ensure safety, efficacy and compatibility with existing medications or health conditions. By exploring alternative approaches to symptom management, women can personalize their care plan according to their values, preferences, and wellness goals during perimenopause.

5.3 Hormone Replacement Therapy (HRT) Options

Hormone Replacement Therapy (HRT) is a common treatment for managing menopausal symptoms. It involves supplementing the body's estrogen and progesterone levels. HRT has been effective in alleviating hot flashes, night sweats, vaginal dryness, mood swings, and other menopausal symptoms. There are various HRT options available to cater to individual needs, preferences, health considerations and treatment goals.

One common form of HRT is systemic estrogen therapy which comes in different forms such as pills, patches, gels, creams, or sprays. It is typically prescribed for women experiencing moderate-to-severe menopausal symptoms such as hot flashes, night sweats, or vaginal dryness. Another type of HRT is low-dose vaginal products, which deliver estrogen directly to the vaginal tissues to alleviate dryness, discomfort, or pain during intercourse.

For women who have undergone hysterectomy (surgical removal of the uterus), estrogen-only therapy may be recommended as there is no need for progestin (synthetic progesterone) to protect against uterine cancer. Combination therapy, which includes both estrogen and progesterone, is often prescribed for women who still have their uterus as progestin helps protect against endometrial cancer caused by unopposed estrogen exposure. Bioidentical hormones, derived from plant sources that are chemically identical to those produced by the body, are another option for HRT that some women may consider due to perceived naturalness or potential benefits over synthetic hormones.

Women considering HRT should discuss the risks, benefits, side effects, and contraindications with healthcare providers before starting treatment. Regular monitoring of hormone levels, symptoms, and overall health status is essential while undergoing HRT to ensure optimal outcomes. By exploring different HRT options available, women can work collaboratively with healthcare providers to find a personalized treatment plan that addresses their unique needs, concerns, and goals.

Navigating perimenopause requires thoughtful consideration of symptom management strategies, treatment options, lifestyle adjustments, and support systems. By taking proactive steps, empowering themselves with knowledge, seeking guidance from healthcare professionals, and building strong networks of support, women can navigate this transformative phase with confidence, resilience, and optimism.

and emotional resilience in the face of hormonal changes.

 It is suggested that incorporating dietary supplements like vitamin D3, calcium or magnesium in the routine can be beneficial for supporting bone health and reducing the risk of osteoporosis associated with declining estrogen levels during perimenopause. However, before including any alternative therapies or natural remedies in the routine, women should consult with healthcare providers to ensure safety, efficacy and compatibility with existing medications or health conditions. By exploring alternative approaches to symptom management, women can personalize their care plan according to their values, preferences, and wellness goals during perimenopause.

5.3 Hormone Replacement Therapy (HRT) Options

 Hormone Replacement Therapy (HRT) is a common treatment for managing menopausal symptoms. It involves supplementing the body's estrogen and progesterone levels. HRT has been effective in alleviating hot flashes, night sweats, vaginal dryness, mood swings, and other menopausal symptoms. There are various HRT options available to cater to individual needs, preferences, health considerations and treatment goals.

One common form of HRT is systemic estrogen therapy which comes in different forms such as pills, patches, gels, creams, or sprays. It is typically prescribed for women experiencing moderate-to-severe menopausal symptoms such as hot flashes, night sweats, or vaginal dryness. Another type of HRT is low-dose vaginal products, which deliver estrogen directly to the vaginal tissues to alleviate dryness, discomfort, or pain during intercourse.

For women who have undergone hysterectomy (surgical removal of the uterus), estrogen-only therapy may be recommended as there is no need for progestin (synthetic progesterone) to protect against uterine cancer. Combination therapy, which includes both estrogen and progesterone, is often prescribed for women who still have their uterus as progestin helps protect against endometrial cancer caused by unopposed estrogen exposure. Bioidentical hormones, derived from plant sources that are chemically identical to those produced by the body, are another option for HRT that some women may consider due to perceived naturalness or potential benefits over synthetic hormones.

Women considering HRT should discuss the risks, benefits, side effects, and contraindications with healthcare providers before starting treatment. Regular monitoring of hormone levels, symptoms, and overall health status is essential while undergoing HRT to ensure optimal outcomes. By exploring different HRT options available, women can work collaboratively with healthcare providers to find a personalized treatment plan that addresses their unique needs, concerns, and goals.

Navigating perimenopause requires thoughtful consideration of symptom management strategies, treatment options, lifestyle adjustments, and support systems. By taking proactive steps, empowering themselves with knowledge, seeking guidance from healthcare professionals, and building strong networks of support, women can navigate this transformative phase with confidence, resilience, and optimism.

Different forms of medication delivery include pills, patches, gels, creams, or sprays. These various methods offer flexibility in how the medication is administered to patients. Pills are a common form that can be easily swallowed with water. Patches provide a slow release of medication through the skin over time. Gels and creams are applied topically to the skin for absorption, while sprays deliver medication through the nasal passages or directly onto affected areas. Each form has its own advantages and may be chosen based on factors such as patient preference, ease of use, or specific medical needs. It is important to follow the instructions provided by healthcare professionals for proper usage and effectiveness of these different forms of medication delivery.

Systemic estrogen therapy is typically prescribed for women experiencing moderate-to-severe menopausal symptoms such as hot flashes, night sweats, or vaginal dryness. Another type of hormone replacement therapy (HRT) involves low-dose vaginal products that deliver estrogen directly to the vaginal tissues. This method helps alleviate dryness, discomfort, and pain during intercourse.

For women who have undergone hysterectomy, estrogen-only therapy may be recommended since there is no need for progestin to protect against uterine cancer. However, for women who still have their uterus, combination therapy with both estrogen and progesterone is often prescribed to prevent endometrial cancer caused by unopposed estrogen exposure. Bioidentical hormones, which are derived from plant sources and chemically identical to those produced by the body, are another option some women may consider for Hormone Replacement Therapy (HRT) due to perceived naturalness or potential benefits over synthetic hormones.

Every woman's journey through perimenopause is distinct and unique. Embracing this chapter with self-compassion, openness, and a positive outlook can empower her to embrace change with grace. With proper care, support, and self-awareness, women can navigate through this transition with ease.

For further reading on perimenopause and menopause, "The Wisdom of Menopause" by Dr. Christiane Northrup offers insights into the physical, emotional, and spiritual aspects of this life stage. Additionally, "Menopause Confidential" by Dr. Tara Allmen provides practical advice on managing symptoms and making informed decisions about treatment options. For evidence-based information, the North American Menopause Society (NAMS) website offers resources and guidelines for women seeking reliable information on menopausal health.

Every woman's journey through perimenopause is as unique as she is. How can you embrace this chapter of your life with self-compassion and openness? What changes are you ready to welcome with open arms? By empowering yourself with a positive mindset, you can navigate through this transition with grace and confidence. Remember, each step you take towards embracing change is a step towards growth and self-discovery. So, are you ready to embrace change and embark on this new chapter of your life with courage and resilience?

For further reading on perimenopause and menopause, "The Wisdom of Menopause" by Dr. Christiane Northrup offers insights into the physical, emotional, and spiritual aspects of this life stage. Additionally, "Menopause Confidential" by Dr. Tara Allmen provides practical advice on managing symptoms and making informed decisions about treatment options. For evidence-based information, the North American Menopause Society (NAMS) website offers resources and guidelines for women seeking reliable information on menopausal health.

Every woman's journey through perimenopause is distinct and unique. Embracing this chapter with self-compassion, openness, and a positive outlook can empower her to embrace change with grace. With proper care, support, and self-awareness, women can navigate through this transition with ease.

For further reading on perimenopause and menopause, "The Wisdom of Menopause" by Dr. Christiane Northrup offers insights into the physical, emotional, and spiritual aspects of this life stage. Additionally, "Menopause Confidential" by Dr. Tara Allmen provides practical advice on managing symptoms and making informed decisions about treatment options. For evidence-based information, the North American Menopause Society (NAMS) website offers resources and guidelines for women seeking reliable information on menopausal health.

Chapter 6: Navigating Relationships and Communication in Perimenopause

6.1 Communicating with Your Partner about Perimenopause

Navigating perimenopause can be a challenging time not only for women but also for their partners. It is essential to communicate openly and honestly about the physical and emotional changes that come with this phase of life. Partners may not always understand what women are going through, so initiating conversations about perimenopausal symptoms, concerns, and needs can foster mutual understanding and support.

Understanding how hot flashes can disrupt sleep or how mood swings can affect daily interactions can provide insight into the challenges faced during perimenopause. It is important to encourage your partner to ask questions and express their own thoughts or concerns in order to create a safe space for dialogue and empathy.

It is crucial to emphasize that perimenopause is a natural biological process and not a choice. Assure your partner that these changes are temporary and part of the journey towards menopause. Setting realistic expectations together can help manage frustrations or misunderstandings that may arise due to hormonal fluctuations.

In some cases, seeking professional guidance from a therapist or counselor specializing in menopausal issues can facilitate communication between partners. These professionals can offer strategies for effective communication, conflict resolution, and mutual support during this transitional phase.

Remember that every relationship is unique, so finding what works best for you and your partner is key. Whether it's scheduling regular check-ins to discuss feelings or exploring new ways to connect emotionally and physically, open communication lays the foundation for navigating perimenopause together as a team.

6.2 Maintaining Healthy Relationships with Family and Friends during Perimenopause

Perimenopause not only impacts women but also those around them, including family members and friends. Maintaining healthy relationships during this time involves open communication, setting boundaries, and seeking support when needed.

Educating family members and friends about perimenopause can help them understand the physical and emotional changes you may be experiencing. By sharing information on common symptoms like hot flashes, mood swings, or fatigue, loved ones can offer empathy and support rather than judgment or misunderstanding.

In some cases, seeking professional guidance from a therapist or counselor specializing in menopausal issues can facilitate communication between partners. These professionals can offer strategies for effective communication, conflict resolution, and mutual support during this transitional phase.

Remember that every relationship is unique, so finding what works best for you and your partner is key. Whether it's scheduling regular check-ins to discuss feelings or exploring new ways to connect emotionally and physically, open communication lays the foundation for navigating perimenopause together as a team.

6.2 Maintaining Healthy Relationships with Family and Friends during Perimenopause

Perimenopause not only impacts women but also those around them, including family members and friends. Maintaining healthy relationships during this time involves open communication, setting boundaries, and seeking support when needed.

Educating family members and friends about perimenopause can help them understand the physical and emotional changes you may be experiencing. By sharing information on common symptoms like hot flashes, mood swings, or fatigue, loved ones can offer empathy and support rather than judgment or misunderstanding.

Healthcare professionals such as gynecologists or endocrinologists can offer personalized treatment options tailored to individual needs based on symptoms severity, medical history, and preferences. They may recommend hormone replacement therapy (HRT), alternative therapies like acupuncture or herbal supplements, or lifestyle modifications to alleviate perimenopausal symptoms effectively.

Support groups dedicated to menopausal women provide a safe space for sharing experiences, seeking advice, and receiving encouragement from others who are going through similar challenges. These groups offer emotional support, empowerment, and companionship that can help combat feelings of isolation or uncertainty often experienced during perimenopause.

When considering treatment options, it's important to consult healthcare providers to ensure safety, effectiveness, and compatibility with existing health conditions or medications. Regular monitoring of symptom progression, hormone levels, and overall health status is crucial while undergoing treatment to optimize outcomes and address any potential concerns promptly.

By proactively seeking support from healthcare professionals and engaging with supportive communities, women navigating perimenopause can feel empowered, informed, and less alone in their journey. Remember that reaching out for help is a sign of strength, not weakness; embracing the resources available ensures you receive comprehensive care and holistic support throughout this transformative phase of life.

Healthcare professionals such as gynecologists or endocrinologists can offer personalized treatment options tailored to individual needs based on symptoms severity, medical history, and preferences. They may recommend hormone replacement therapy (HRT), alternative therapies like acupuncture or herbal supplements, or lifestyle modifications to alleviate perimenopausal symptoms effectively.

Support groups dedicated to menopausal women provide a safe space for sharing experiences, seeking advice, and receiving encouragement from others who are going through similar challenges. These groups offer emotional support, empowerment, and companionship that can help combat feelings of isolation or uncertainty often experienced during perimenopause.

When considering treatment options, it's important to consult healthcare providers to ensure safety, effectiveness, and compatibility with existing health conditions or medications. Regular monitoring of symptom progression, hormone levels, and overall health status is crucial while undergoing treatment to optimize outcomes and address any potential concerns promptly.

 By proactively seeking support from healthcare professionals and engaging with supportive communities, women navigating perimenopause can feel empowered, informed, and less alone in their journey. Remember that reaching out for help is a sign of strength, not weakness; embracing the resources available ensures you receive comprehensive care and holistic support throughout this transformative phase of life.

 In conclusion, openly communicating with your partner, maintaining healthy relationships with family and friends, seeking guidance from healthcare professionals, and joining support groups are vital components of navigating perimenopause successfully. By prioritizing effective communication, setting boundaries, seeking professional advice, and connecting with supportive communities, women can embrace this transition with resilience, confidence, and optimism. They can navigate this transformative stage with grace, dignity, and strength by knowing they have the tools, resources, and support systems in place.

Navigating perimenopause with grace and strength involves prioritizing open communication and embracing change for personal growth and well-being. Joining online support groups like Menopause Chicks or MyMenopauseTeam can connect you with a community of women going through similar experiences, providing mutual support during this transformative phase of life.

Remember to consult healthcare professionals for personalized advice and treatment options tailored to your specific needs. Stay informed, connected, and empowered as you navigate perimenopause. Embracing change and seeking support will help you navigate this unique journey with resilience and positivity

and overall health status is crucial while undergoing treatment to optimize outcomes and address any potential concerns promptly.

By proactively seeking support from healthcare professionals and engaging with supportive communities, women navigating perimenopause can feel empowered, informed, and less alone in their journey. Remember that reaching out for help is a sign of strength, not weakness; embracing the resources available ensures you receive comprehensive care and holistic support throughout this transformative phase of life.

In conclusion, communicating openly with your partner, maintaining healthy relationships with family and friends, seeking guidance from healthcare professionals, and support groups are vital components of navigating perimenopause successfully. By prioritizing effective communication, setting boundaries, seeking professional advice, and connecting with supportive communities, women can embrace this transition with resilience, confidence, and optimism. Knowing they have the tools, resources, and support systems in place to navigate this transformative stage with grace, dignity, and strength. Each woman's journey through perimenopause is unique but by embracing change.

and overall health status is crucial while undergoing treatment to optimize outcomes and address any potential concerns promptly.

By proactively seeking support from healthcare professionals and engaging with supportive communities, women navigating perimenopause can feel empowered, informed, and less alone in their journey. Remember that reaching out for help is a sign of strength, not weakness; embracing the resources available ensures you receive comprehensive care and holistic support throughout this transformative phase of life.

In conclusion, communicating openly with your partner, maintaining healthy relationships with family and friends, seeking guidance from healthcare professionals, and support groups are vital components of navigating perimenopause successfully. By prioritizing effective communication, setting boundaries, seeking professional advice, and connecting with supportive communities, women can embrace this transition with resilience, confidence, and optimism. Knowing they have the tools, resources, and support systems in place to navigate this transformative stage with grace, dignity, and strength. Each woman's journey through perimenopause is unique but by embracing change.

Joining online support groups such as Menopause Chicks (https://www.menopausechicks.com) or MyMenopauseTeam (https://www.mymenopauseteam.com) can connect you with a community of women sharing similar experiences and offering mutual support.

Remember to consult with healthcare professionals for personalized advice and treatment options tailored to your specific needs during perimenopause. Stay informed, connected, and empowered as you navigate this transformative phase of life.

Synopsis: "What in the Perimenopause is this!" is a comprehensive guide that explores the often misunderstood phase of perimenopause. The book delves into the physical, emotional, and mental changes that women experience during this transitional period, offering practical advice on managing symptoms, seeking medical support, and embracing self-care practices.

Key topics covered in the book include symptoms of perimenopause such as hot flashes, mood swings, hormonal fluctuations, and fertility concerns. It also discusses strategies for managing these symptoms through hormone replacement therapy, lifestyle adjustments, and proactive healthcare decision-making. The book emphasizes the importance of self-awareness, self-compassion, and informed choices in navigating perimenopause.

Notable insights presented in the book include real-life stories and experiences from women going through perimenopause, providing a relatable perspective for readers. The book aims to empower women to advocate for their health and well-being during this transformative time by breaking down complex medical information into digestible insights.

Overall, "What in the Perimenopause is this!" serves as a valuable resource for anyone interested in understanding and navigating the complexities of midlife hormonal changes. It offers a blend of research-based information, personal anecdotes, and practical tips to guide readers through perimenopause with resilience and grace.